FELDENKRAIS METHOD

A Comprehensive Guide To The Feldenkrais Method For Mindful Movement, Pain Relief, And Lifelong Well-Being

WILFREDO CARSON

pg. 1

INTRODUCTION

The Feldenkrais Method is a somatic educational technique aimed at increasing self-awareness and improving movement patterns. Dr. Moshe Feldenkrais, a physicist and judo specialist, developed this system, which combines physics, biomechanics, and neurology to encourage efficient and effortless movement. The next lines discuss the Feldenkrais Method's history and origins, as well as its purpose and scope, and offer advice on how to utilize it effectively.

<u>Background & Origins of the Feldenkrais Method:</u>

Dr. Moshe Feldenkrais' diversified skills led to the development of the Feldenkrais Method. Feldenkrais, born in 1904, encountered physical obstacles early in life, prompting him to experiment with numerous movement modalities before developing his method.

His education in physics and engineering, as well as his judo training, informed the Feldenkrais Method's distinct set of underlying principles. Feldenkrais aimed to build a comprehensive method that addressed both the physical and neurological components of movement, to improve flexibility, coordination, and overall health. Over time, the approach has evolved and garnered a reputation for its efficacy in increasing body awareness and encouraging healthy movement patterns.

<u>Purpose and Scope of the Book:</u>

This comprehensive handbook seeks to provide a thorough understanding of the concepts that underpin the Feldenkrais Method. Its goal is to provide readers with a comprehensive grasp of the principles and practices that underpin this somatic approach. By delving into the method's complexities, the book aims to be a beneficial resource for those looking to expand their understanding of body-mind connections, movement optimization, and holistic well-being. The book goes beyond a basic review, diving into the complexities of the Feldenkrais Method, its applicability in many circumstances, and the potential advantages for people of all ages and abilities.

<u>How To Use This Guide:</u>

To properly traverse this guide, readers should approach it as a progressive investigation of the Feldenkrais Method.

The information is designed to provide a solid basis for knowledge before moving on to more advanced subjects. Begin by learning about the method's history and beginnings, acquiring an understanding of Dr. Moshe Feldenkrais' multidisciplinary approach. As you proceed, the guide will explain the fundamental concepts of the Feldenkrais Method, offering a framework for understanding its applications in movement instruction and rehabilitation. Practical tasks and examples will be incorporated throughout the guide to help readers understand and learn via experience. To get the most out of this book, readers should actively engage with the information, applying the ideas to their own movement experiences and thinking about the potential impact on their well-being.

<u>Body of the Guide:</u>

The Feldenkrais Method is based on the core principle of neuroplasticity, which emphasizes the brain's ability to restructure itself in response to novel experiences and learning. Individuals engage in self-discovery through gentle and exploratory movements, which promotes increased awareness and functional movement. This section digs into important concepts at the heart of the Feldenkrais Method, providing insights into its applicability in a variety of areas.

<u>Awareness via Movement (ATM):</u>

Awareness Through Movement (ATM) is one of the key ways in which people connect with the Feldenkrais Method. These sessions are intended to lead learners through a sequence of mindful movements that promote exploration and self-awareness.

The emphasis is not on reaching specific goals, but on developing a better understanding of one's body and movement patterns. Individuals can break free from typical habits and discover more efficient ways of moving by focusing on minor nuances of feeling.

ATM classes cover a wide range of tasks, from simple processes like breathing and sitting to more complicated ones like walking or reaching. This section delves into the fundamentals of ATM, emphasizing its function in fostering neuroplasticity, increasing kinesthetic awareness, and supporting beneficial movement patterns.

Functional Integration (Fi):

Functional Integration (FI) is the hands-on part of the Feldenkrais Method in which a practitioner works one-on-one with a client. The practitioner delivers input to the client's neurological system via gentle and non-invasive touch, resulting in a greater sense of self-awareness. FI sessions are adjusted to the individual's unique demands and movement patterns, with the goal of establishing optimal conditions for learning and discovery.

This section goes into the concepts of FI, looking at the role of tactile feedback, the value of tailored sessions, and how movement education may be integrated into the client's general well-being. The comprehensive nature of FI highlights its ability to treat not just physical constraints, but also the emotional and cognitive aspects of a person's experience.

<u>Principles of Motion and Function:</u>

The Feldenkrais Method is based on principles that govern the investigation and comprehension of movement.

These ideas are derived from anatomy, biomechanics, and the overall concept of neuroplasticity. Individuals can acquire insights into improving movement efficiency and reducing strain or injury by studying the interaction of the neurological system, skeletal structure, and muscle coordination.

This section discusses fundamental notions such as reversibility, differentiation, and the importance of purpose in movement. Understanding these principles gives people a framework for applying Feldenkrais concepts beyond specific courses, incorporating them into daily activities, and cultivating a more aware and flexible approach to movement.

<u>Integration in Daily Life:</u>

The Feldenkrais Method's ultimate purpose is to help people integrate improved movement patterns into their daily lives. This entails going beyond the scope of formal instruction and applying the ideas of awareness and functional improvement to a variety of activities. Whether sitting at a computer, walking, or participating in sports, individuals can use the insights garnered from the approach to improve their overall well-being. This part delves into practical Feldenkrais Method applications in a variety of scenarios, with a focus on the transferability of knowledge gained during ATM and FI sessions to real-world situations.

The integration process goes beyond physical motions to include emotional resilience, stress reduction, and cognitive adaptability. Individuals can reap long-term advantages and continue to find themselves by incorporating Feldenkrais's ideas into their daily lives.

Applications for Rehabilitation and Performance Enhancement:

The Feldenkrais Method has been recognized for its use in rehabilitation and performance development in a variety of sectors. This section looks at how the approach is used to help people heal from accidents, manage chronic diseases, and improve their performance in sports and the arts. The guide uses case studies and examples to demonstrate how the Feldenkrais Method can be applied to a wide range of demographics and settings. Whether dealing with athletes, musicians, or those with neurological disorders, the method's emphasis on customized and exploratory learning is effective in promoting positive outcomes. Understanding the subtle application of the Feldenkrais Method in rehabilitation and performance situations allows practitioners to adjust their approach to their client's specific requirements.

<u>Research and Evidence Base:</u>

As interest in complementary and alternative approaches to health and well-being rises, the Feldenkrais Method has been a focus of research in a variety of fields. This section examines previous research and the evidence supporting the method's effectiveness.

The guide includes an overview of the current research landscape, including studies measuring its impact on chronic pain and examinations of neuroplastic changes connected with Feldenkrais practice. Furthermore, it identifies areas where more research is needed to better understand the mechanisms underlying the method's good impacts. By critically reviewing the data foundation, practitioners and researchers can help shape and validate the Feldenkrais Method in the scientific and healthcare sectors.

The Feldenkrais Method is a holistic and transformative approach to movement education and self-awareness. Based on Dr. Moshe Feldenkrais' extensive skills, the approach has evolved into a holistic paradigm that addresses body-mind interdependence.

This guide provides a road map for those interested in learning more about the Feldenkrais Method's underlying ideas and practices. From the fundamental principles of neuroplasticity and awareness through movement to the hands-on aspect of functional integration, the guide delves deeply into the method's major components. Individuals who embrace the ideas stated in this guide can start on a journey of self-discovery, improved well-being, and a deeper understanding of their body's capacity for adaptable and efficient movement.

CHAPTER 1
THE FOUNDATIONS OF THE FELDENKRAIS METHOD

<u>Understanding Moshe Feldenkrais.</u>

Moshe Feldenkrais, the originator of the Feldenkrais Method, was a multidimensional individual with knowledge in a multitude of subjects. He was born in Ukraine in 1904 and went on to become a scientist, engineer, judo specialist, and accomplished martial artist. Feldenkrais traveled from Eastern Europe to Paris, where he got a Ph.D. in Engineering and had a strong interest in the relationships between movement, learning, and healing. His broad background and experiences had a significant impact on the development of the Feldenkrais Method, which he created in response to his personal knee ailment.

Feldenkrais's understanding of neuroplasticity, the brain's ability to rearrange itself, became a cornerstone of his method, demonstrating the potential for individuals to increase their physical and mental well-being through intentional movement and awareness.

<u>Principles and Philosophy:</u>

The Feldenkrais Method is founded on a set of principles and beliefs that govern its practice and use. One such notion is the emphasis on the innate ability to self-improve. Feldenkrais thought that individuals could improve their functioning and well-being through a process of self-discovery and inquiry. This idea is consistent with the concept of neuroplasticity, which states that the brain can change and restructure itself in response to new experiences.

Another important element is understanding the interdependence of the mind and body. Feldenkrais saw the movement as a way to comprehend and influence cognitive and emotional states. Individuals who cultivate awareness of their movements might have a better understanding of their habits and patterns, which leads to improved self-regulation.

<u>Awareness through Movement:</u>

The Feldenkrais Method is built around the practice of Awareness Through Movement (ATM). ATM comprises guided movement courses that aim to raise self-awareness and improve general functioning. A practitioner verbally guides these teachings, urging participants to experiment with different movements, pay attention to feelings, and make tiny adjustments.

The emphasis is on quality rather than quantity of movement, with people encouraged to move within their comfort zones and investigate the relationships between various areas of their bodies. ATM teaches participants to pay conscious attention to their motions, which promotes self-discovery and allows for the refinement of habitual patterns.

The overarching goal is to improve flexibility, coordination, and well-being.

<u>Functional integration:</u>

In addition to Awareness Through Movement, the Feldenkrais Method includes Functional Integration (FI). Unlike ATM, FI consists of one-on-one sessions in which a practitioner uses hands-on, soft touch to guide the client's movements.

These sessions are personalized to the individual's specific requirements and limitations, with the practitioner employing expert touch and verbal cues to help the client become aware of and explore movement possibilities. Functional Integration strives to address individual concerns or limits, delivering a targeted and nuanced approach to improve overall function. Practitioners who provide individualized attention can alter their techniques to match the client's specific goals, creating a greater level of self-awareness and promoting good changes in movement patterns.

<u>Mind-Body Connection:</u>

The Feldenkrais Method emphasizes the delicate link between the mind and body. Moshe Feldenkrais observed that our ideas, emotions, and physical movements are inextricably linked, influencing one another in a continual feedback loop.

ATM and FI encourage people to intentionally examine the mind-body link. Participants get insights into their cognitive processes and emotional responses by increasing their awareness of movement and the sensations that accompany it. This increased awareness can improve both physical functioning and mental well-being.

Thus, the Feldenkrais Method is a comprehensive approach that recognizes the interdependence of the mental and physical dimensions of human experience.

The Feldenkrais Method's historical evolution can be traced back to Moshe Feldenkrais' path of self-discovery and healing. After suffering a knee injury, Feldenkrais began researching various movement patterns and strategies to regain his mobility. This investigation created the groundwork for what would eventually become the Feldenkrais Method.

The system evolved when Feldenkrais combined his expertise in physics, engineering, and martial arts with ideas from neurology and psychology. Feldenkrais' early Judo instruction inspired his method's emphasis on soft, non-forceful movements. Over time, the practice acquired popularity and acceptance in Europe and North America, drawing those looking for alternatives to standard movement and rehabilitation techniques.

As the Feldenkrais Method expanded, it was further refined and adapted. Several practitioners and trainers helped shape its progress, adding new ideas and ways while adhering to its essential principles.

The method's versatility has allowed it to be used in a variety of sectors, including performing arts, athletics, rehabilitation, and wellness. The Feldenkrais Method is still evolving today thanks to ongoing research, training programs, and the incorporation of cutting-edge knowledge in neuroscience and somatic education. Its historical history indicates a dedication to continual improvement and a willingness to adapt to the changing requirements of people trying to improve their physical and mental health.

The Feldenkrais Method is founded on Moshe Feldenkrais' life and experiences, driven by concepts and philosophies that emphasize self-improvement, the mind-body link, and neuroplasticity. The combination of Awareness Through Movement and Functional Integration creates a complete approach to movement education and rehabilitation. The method's historical growth emphasizes its adaptability and continuous evolution, making it a beneficial and dynamic way to improve human potential and well-being.

CHAPTER 2

CORE PRINCIPLES OF AWARENESS THROUGH MOVEMENT

The Feldenkrais Method, created by Moshe Feldenkrais, is based on the key concepts of Awareness Through Movement.

These concepts serve as the method's foundation, emphasizing the relationship between mind and body, as well as movement and awareness. Individuals engage in exploratory movements as part of a series of planned classes to increase their self-awareness and well-being.

Exploring Awareness Through Movement Lessons.

The Feldenkrais Method places a strong emphasis on investigating Awareness Through Movement (ATM) principles.

These classes include gentle movements and body awareness activities that aim to improve a person's perception of their own body and movement patterns. The emphasis on gentleness is critical since it aligns with Feldenkrais' view that delicate, non-habitual motions can result in large increases in awareness and flexibility. Participants are urged to move gently and with curiosity, focusing on their bodies' sensations and input.

Gentle Movement and Body Awareness

The Feldenkrais Method differs from more traditional workout programs in that it emphasizes gentle movements during Awareness Through Movement lessons.

The rationale for gentle motions stems from the assumption that aggressive or sudden acts can elicit defensive responses, impeding the learning process. Individuals can explore new possibilities by moving slowly and deliberately, avoiding habitual patterns and unnecessary strain. This emphasis on gentleness encourages a conscious approach to movement, resulting in a stronger connection between the mind and body.

The Function of Attention and Intention

The Feldenkrais Method emphasizes the complex interplay between attention and purpose in movement. Participants are encouraged to be more mindful of their motions, focusing on quality rather than quantity. Individuals can uncover new possibilities for efficient and harmonious behaviors by focusing on the nuances of movement and experimenting with different intentions. This intentional approach is consistent with the Feldenkrais Method's overall philosophy, which emphasizes the need for mindful engagement in the learning process.

<u>Breathing Techniques</u>

Awareness Through Movement lessons frequently include particular breathing methods to increase overall awareness and well-being. Feldenkrais realized that breath plays an important role in movement and emotional states. Participants can gain a better understanding of how breath affects movement patterns and overall body function by introducing conscious breathing into their sessions.

pg. 28

The addition of breath work expands the Feldenkrais Method's holistic approach, addressing not just physical movement but also the interconnected components of mental and emotional well-being.

Applying Feldenkrais' Principles to Daily Life

Beyond organized classes, the Feldenkrais Method has a broader impact on daily living, including practical applications of its principles to improve general functioning.

The goal is to incorporate the knowledge obtained from Awareness Through Movement sessions into daily activities, thereby improving posture, movement efficiency, and overall well-being.

<u>Sitting and standing with ease.</u>

One application of Feldenkrais concepts in daily life is to sit and stand comfortably.

Many people feel discomfort or stress during these seemingly easy activities as a result of regular movement patterns or poor posture. Feldenkrais aims to address these concerns by raising awareness of how people interact with sitting and standing. Individuals can learn to distribute their weight more efficiently, eliminate unneeded tension, and establish a more comfortable and lasting relationship with these essential postures by exploring and adjusting gently.

<u>Efficient walking and movement patterns.</u>

The Feldenkrais Method also emphasizes creating efficient walking and movement patterns to improve daily functioning. Individuals who apply the principles of Awareness Through Movement to walking can improve their gait, balance, and overall coordination.

This includes investigating changes in stride length, foot location, and the subtleties of weight transfer while walking. The goal is to build a more balanced, fluid, and energy-efficient manner of moving, applying Feldenkrais principles to everyday activities.

The Feldenkrais Method's Core Principles of Awareness Through Movement serve as a comprehensive framework for investigating the complex link between mind and body.

The emphasis on gentle movements, attention, intention, and breathing methods in structured courses sets the groundwork for greater self-awareness and well-being. Furthermore, applying Feldenkrais principles to daily living, such as sitting and standing comfortably or establishing efficient walking patterns, broadens the benefits beyond the constraints of a lesson, fostering a holistic approach to movement and mindfulness.

CHAPTER 3
FUNCTIONAL INTEGRATION: A PERSONALIZED APPROACH

An overview of functional integration sessions:

Functional Integration is a core idea in the Feldenkrais Method, which emphasizes a tailored and hands-on approach to improving an individual's awareness and movement patterns. In Functional Integration sessions, practitioners work one-on-one with clients, personalizing each session to their specific requirements and concerns. These sessions are distinguished by a thorough examination of movement, with a particular emphasis on improving overall coordination. The goal is to increase self-awareness and improve general function through gentle, non-invasive touch and vocal direction.

Functional Integration sessions usually begin with the practitioner monitoring the client's movement patterns and determining their range of motion. Practitioners detect regions of restriction or inefficiency by paying close attention and studying biomechanics.

The emphasis is on movement quality rather than quantity, and the lessons are meant to help students learn through sensory-motor experiences. Functional Integration attempts to increase physical well-being for the long term by addressing underlying movement patterns and fostering more effective ways of doing daily activities.

Hands-on Techniques and Gentle Manipulation:

pg. 34

Practitioners' use of hands-on techniques and gentle manipulations is critical to the effectiveness of Functional Integration sessions. Practitioners use a combination of touch, movement, and verbal coaching to elicit heightened awareness in the client, allowing for a thorough examination of their movement potential. The touch utilized in Functional Integration is sensitive and precise, with soft, non-invasive manipulations that stimulate the nervous system and encourage relaxation.

<u>Working with the nervous system:</u>

Functional integration recognizes the complex relationship between movement and the neurological system. Practitioners use touch and movement to connect with the neurological system, hoping to elicit tiny changes in muscle tone, coordination, and general body awareness. The mild manipulations aim to stimulate the proprioceptive and kinesthetic senses, resulting in a more refined understanding of one's own body and movement. Functional Integration works with the neurological system to generate new neural pathways, allowing for more efficient and adaptive movement patterns.

<u>Customizing Sessions to Meet Individual Needs:</u>

One of Functional Integration's primary features is its capacity to be highly tailored. Each session is tailored to the client's individual needs and goals. Practitioners consider the client's individual movement patterns, limits, and areas of discomfort.

Sessions are customized by modifying hands-on techniques, movement explorations, and verbal prompts to the individual's specific issues. This tailored method enables more targeted and effective instruction, encouraging optimal learning and improvement in movement patterns.

<u>Integrating Mind-Body Harmony.</u>

Functional Integration extends beyond the physical characteristics of movement to include the concept of mind-body harmony. The method acknowledges the interdependence of physical, emotional, and cognitive aspects of an individual's life. Practitioners strive to provide the client with a complete and integrated experience by using hands-on approaches and individualized sessions. This integration entails not just improved physical movement, but also a greater awareness of one's thoughts, emotions, and overall health.

Functional Integration promotes mind-body harmony via mindful movement exploration and the development of conscious, nonjudgmental awareness. Throughout the sessions, clients are urged to focus on their sensations, thoughts, and feelings.

This increased awareness enables a deeper grasp of the relationships between physical activity and mental moods. By integrating the mind-body connection, Functional Integration seeks to promote a sense of balance, resilience, and well-being in individuals.

Functional Integration in the Feldenkrais Method provides a tailored and nuanced approach to enhancing movement patterns and general well-being. Its hands-on techniques, personalized sessions, and emphasis on mind-body harmony make it a thorough and successful approach to increasing self-awareness and encouraging optimal functioning. Functional Integration enables people to explore and optimize their movement potential through mild manipulations and a thorough grasp of the neurological system, resulting in long-term gains in physical and mental health.

CHAPTER 4
THE BENEFITS OF PRACTICING THE FELDENKRAIS METHOD

The Feldenkrais Method is a somatic educational approach that focuses on improving movement and overall well-being by increasing self-awareness and attention to the body. Moshe Feldenkrais developed this method, which uses gentle, mindful movements to promote self-discovery while also improving physical and mental functioning. In this discussion, we will look at the benefits of practicing the Feldenkrais Method, including physical and emotional/mental well-being.

<u>Physical Wellbeing</u>

Pain Relief and Rehabilitation One of the key benefits of practicing the Feldenkrais Method is the reduction of pain and support in rehabilitation. Through a sequence of slow, purposeful motions, individuals can gain a heightened awareness of their bodies, detecting areas of tension and discomfort.

The technique encourages a non-judgmental examination of these experiences, enabling self-correction and improved movement patterns. By addressing the root causes of pain, Feldenkrais contributes to pain relief and aids in the rehabilitation process. This is particularly beneficial for individuals recovering from injuries or dealing with chronic pain conditions.

Enhancing Flexibility and Coordination

The Feldenkrais Method places a strong emphasis on improving flexibility and coordination. Through its unique combination of movements and heightened body awareness, individuals can explore new ways of moving, expanding their range of motion. The method encourages gentle and precise actions that aim to break habitual patterns and create more efficient and coordinated movements. Over time, this can lead to increased flexibility, better posture, and improved overall physical performance. Whether applied in sports, daily activities, or specific therapeutic contexts, the method's focus on enhancing flexibility and coordination contributes to an individual's physical well-being.

Emotional and Mental Well-being

Stress Reduction and Relaxation Beyond its physical benefits, the Feldenkrais Method has a profound impact on emotional and mental well-being. The practice involves gentle, mindful movements that induce a state of deep relaxation. By guiding individuals to pay attention to their breath, movements, and sensations, the method promotes a heightened sense of awareness and presence. This mindful approach contributes to stress reduction, helping individuals release tension and find a more centered state of being. The emphasis on relaxation in Feldenkrais can be particularly valuable in today's fast-paced and stressful environments, offering a holistic approach to well-being.

Improved Cognitive Function The Feldenkrais Method is not solely focused on the body; it also recognizes the intricate connection between body and mind.

Through its emphasis on mindful movement and heightened awareness, the method positively influences cognitive function.

The intricate interplay between movement and thought processes is explored in a non-linear and exploratory manner. This unique approach can lead to improved cognitive abilities, such as enhanced focus, concentration, and problem-solving skills. By holistically engaging both body and mind, the Feldenkrais Method provides a comprehensive approach to improving overall mental well-being.

In summary, the Feldenkrais Method offers a multifaceted approach to well-being, encompassing both physical and emotional/mental aspects. Through its emphasis on mindful movement, heightened awareness, and non-judgmental exploration, individuals can experience pain relief, rehabilitation, enhanced flexibility, coordination, stress reduction, relaxation, and improved cognitive function. As a holistic and integrative method, Feldenkrais stands as a valuable tool for those seeking to cultivate a deeper connection with their bodies and promote overall well-being.

CHAPTER 5
INTEGRATING FELDENKRAIS INTO YOUR LIFESTYLE

The Feldenkrais Method, established by Moshe Feldenkrais, is a holistic approach to movement and self-awareness. This practice stresses the connection between mind and body, seeking to promote movement efficiency, flexibility, and overall well-being. Integrating Feldenkrais into one's lifestyle means adapting its concepts into daily activities, work, ergonomics, exercise, fitness, and establishing a personal practice routine. This comprehensive approach offers a unique perspective on enhancing the quality of movement and promoting mindfulness in various aspects of life.

Incorporating Feldenkrais concepts into daily tasks is a crucial component of embracing this system. By employing the concepts of awareness, focus, and intention, individuals can transform regular behaviors into chances for self-discovery and progress. Mindful movement becomes a fundamental aspect in tasks like walking, sitting, and even simple motions. This heightened awareness can lead to increased comfort, lower tension, and improved general functionality in day-to-day tasks.

Work and ergonomics play a key part in the integration of Feldenkrais concepts.

The strategy stresses developing ergonomic workspaces and cultivating efficient movement patterns to reduce strain and damage. By applying Feldenkrais concepts to work activities, individuals can strengthen their posture, reduce tension, and optimize their physical well-being while executing tasks. This not only aids in physical health but also increases mental clarity and concentration during work-related activities.

Exercise and fitness are areas where the Feldenkrais Method can make a major influence. Instead of focusing entirely on standard workout routines, combining Feldenkrais concepts into fitness activities can lead to a more conscious and balanced approach. This involves paying attention to the quality of movement, exploring different variants, and customizing routines to fit individual needs. By doing so, individuals can feel greater flexibility, coordination, and a heightened sense of physiological awareness during physical activity.

Building a personal practice routine is a fundamental component of incorporating Feldenkrais into one's lifestyle. Designing an Awareness Through Movement (ATM) routine allows individuals to personalize their practice to unique needs and goals. This involves a sequence of guided motions that develop self-awareness and increased function. Creating a routine that matches personal preferences and areas of progress enables individuals to adopt Feldenkrais principles into their daily lives in a sustainable and meaningful way.

The process of designing an ATM routine entails selecting movements that target specific areas of the body or address particular needs. It could entail experimenting with different movements and gradually graduating to more complex sequences. The emphasis is on moving with awareness, paying attention to sensations, and making little adjustments to improve the overall quality of movement. Individuals can have a better understanding of their bodies and learn to move more easily and efficiently with regular practice.

Exploring Functional Integration exercises is another aspect of developing a personal practice routine using the Feldenkrais method. Unlike ATM, Functional Integration (FI) entails one-on-one sessions with a trained practitioner who employs gentle touch and verbal assistance to help people improve their movement patterns. These individualized sessions address specific concerns or limits, adapting the experience to the individual's exact needs. Individuals who include FI in their routines might benefit from tailored coaching and instruction to improve their overall movement capabilities.

Integrating the Feldenkrais Method into one's life requires a diverse approach. Individuals who incorporate its ideas into their everyday activities, work, ergonomics, exercise, and fitness might see a significant improvement in their overall well-being. Building a personal practice routine, which includes creating an ATM program and experimenting with Functional Integration exercises, gives an organized and individualized framework for implementing Feldenkrais principles into daily life. Individuals can cultivate a stronger connection between mind and body through these techniques, resulting in improved movement, increased self-awareness, and a greater sense of overall vitality.

CHAPTER 6: ADVANCED APPLICATIONS AND SPECIALIZED AREAS

Feldenkrais for specific populations.

The Feldenkrais Method has proven to be a diverse and successful strategy for addressing the specific needs of different groups. Children and individuals pursuing developmental education are one such category. In this case, the method's emphasis on soft, exploratory movements and increased awareness is especially useful. The Feldenkrais technique promotes optimum neurodevelopment by helping children refine motor skills, improve coordination, and promote overall physical and cognitive development. Through the use of play and guided movements, practitioners tailor the method to meet the developmental phases of children, offering a comprehensive approach to supporting their progress.

Athletes and sports performance are another area where the Feldenkrais Method has gained traction. Athletes can enhance their overall performance while also lowering their risk of injury by focusing on improving movement patterns and enhancing body awareness.

The method's emphasis on efficient and smooth movement enables athletes to optimize their biomechanics, increase flexibility, and improve coordination. This not only improves athletic performance but also helps with injury prevention and rehabilitation. Feldenkrais becomes an invaluable resource for athletes looking to optimize their ability while maintaining a healthy, sustainable practice in their particular sports.

The Feldenkrais Method provides elders with a holistic approach to aging gracefully. As people age, maintaining mobility, balance, and cognitive function becomes increasingly vital. Feldenkrais offers a gentle and non-intrusive approach to treating these difficulties.

Seniors can regain or retain their capacity to move freely and confidently by engaging in mindful movement exploration and increasing body awareness. Because of its versatility, the approach may be adjusted to seniors' unique needs and talents, making it an important tool for boosting general well-being in the aging population.

Complementary Approaches and Integrations

Feldenkrais and Yoga share a focus on movement, breath awareness, and mindfulness.

Integrating these two methods can produce a synergistic impact, maximizing the benefits of both modalities. The Feldenkrais Method emphasizes gentle, exploratory movements that complement yoga's more organized and static postures.

Individuals who incorporate Feldenkrais principles into their yoga practice can increase body awareness, refine movement patterns, and improve general flexibility and coordination. This integration takes a holistic approach to physical well-being, incorporating the benefits of both modalities to provide a more thorough and customized practice.

Similarly, combining Feldenkrais and meditation creates an effective mix of movement awareness and mental attention. While meditation has historically involved silence and mental concentration, Feldenkrais adds a dynamic aspect with gentle, exploratory movements.

This convergence enables people to have a greater awareness of both their bodies and their minds. Feldenkrais principles can help practitioners improve their meditation practice by fostering a stronger sense of embodiment and ease in silence.

This combination offers a unique opportunity for people to deepen their meditation experience while also embracing movement as a complementing component of mindfulness.

The Feldenkrais Method's expanded applications and specialized areas demonstrate its adaptability and effectiveness across a wide range of demographics and settings. From addressing children's developmental needs to improving athlete performance, promoting graceful aging in seniors, and seamlessly integrating with practices such as yoga and meditation, the Feldenkrais Method continues to demonstrate its versatility as a holistic approach to movement and well-being.

CHAPTER 7
FUTURE DIRECTIONS AND CONTINUOUS LEARNING

The Feldenkrais Method, which takes a comprehensive approach to movement and self-awareness, has grown in popularity in recent years. As practitioners and enthusiasts explore further its concepts and applications, the area is primed for expansion and advancement. Ongoing research is an important part of this trajectory since it not only verifies existing techniques but also allows for refinement and innovation. Researchers are looking into the neuroscientific foundations of the Feldenkrais Method, hoping to gain a better understanding of how the brain and body interact throughout the practice.

pg. 58

The combination of sophisticated technology, like as neuroimaging and biomechanical analysis, represents a viable avenue for resolving the complexities of this strategy.

The Feldenkrais Method's confluence with different fields is another area of future research. Collaborations with sectors such as psychology, sports science, and rehabilitation medicine may provide useful insights into the method's larger applicability. Understanding how Feldenkrais Method principles complement and enhance other therapeutic methods may open the road for multidisciplinary interventions. Furthermore, ongoing studies may reveal certain populations or situations that can greatly benefit from this strategy, broadening its scope and influence.

Training and Certification for the Feldenkrais Method

As the Feldenkrais Method gains popularity, there is a greater need for standardized training and certification. Training programs that are already in place provide an organized curriculum to students desiring to become certified practitioners. These classes cover the method's theoretical foundations, movement-related anatomy and physiology, and practical applications through hands-on experience.

The certification procedure normally consists of coursework, practical tests, and supervised teaching experiences.

Quality assurance and accreditation systems are critical for ensuring the Feldenkrais

Method's integrity as it acquires widespread awareness.

Professional groups and institutions play an important role in developing and maintaining these standards. Ongoing discourse and collaboration among trained practitioners, educators, and accrediting agencies are critical for improving and upgrading training programs to reflect changing understandings of movement science and neuroplasticity.

Continuing education for credentialed practitioners is similarly important. Advanced training modules, workshops, and mentorship programs enable practitioners to expand their knowledge and enhance their abilities.

This continuing learning ensures that practitioners are up to date on the latest advances in the industry and are always improving their ability to enable transformative experiences for their clients. Furthermore, establishing a professional network that promotes peer learning and knowledge sharing helps the Feldenkrais Method grow and mature over time.

Community and Resources for Further Exploration

The Feldenkrais Method's long-term success is built on a sense of community among its practitioners and enthusiasts. As the technique gets popularity, the formation of strong communities provides a forum for sharing experiences, thoughts, and resources. Online forums, social media groups, and local meet-ups encourage networking and collaboration, building a sense of belonging among people who are committed to the practice.

These communities work as information centers, providing a dynamic forum for debating best practices, case studies, and developing research.

Resources for further investigation include a diverse range of information intended to help both novices and seasoned practitioners. Books, articles, and online courses dive into the theoretical basis of the Feldenkrais Method, providing detailed insights into its philosophy and applications. Video demos and guided activities offer visual and experiential learning possibilities, appealing to a variety of learning styles. Furthermore, curated libraries of research articles and publications contribute to the field's academic rigor, bridging the theoretical and practical divide.

Continued collaboration and resource sharing among diverse communities, whether geographical or interest-based, enriches the collective knowledge base.

Local study groups, workshops, and worldwide conferences provide opportunities for practitioners to network, share their experiences, and have meaningful discussions. These interactions contribute to the evolution of the Feldenkrais Method, promoting a culture of constant improvement and innovation.

CONCLUSION

The Feldenkrais Method, which combines neuroscience, movement science, and holistic well-being, provides a unique approach to self-awareness and increased functioning.

Its principles, based on the concept of neuroplasticity, emphasize the brain's adaptability and the possibility of lifelong learning and development. The method's emphasis on conscious movement, improved proprioception, and building a deeper connection between the mind and body has sparked interest in a variety of sectors, including rehabilitation, performing arts, and personal development.

The Feldenkrais Method's future appears hopeful, with continuous research aimed at uncovering its neuroscientific processes and its uses in a variety of scenarios. Standardized training and certification systems assure the method's integrity and quality while continuing education options help practitioners improve professionally. Community-building initiatives, both online and offline, generate a supportive network for information exchange and collaboration, instilling a sense of shared purpose among people committed to the technique.

As the Feldenkrais Method evolves, it can bridge the gap between traditional approaches to movement and new understandings of the mind-body link. Its holistic approach, based on Moshe Feldenkrais' philosophy, appeals to anyone looking for not only physical development but also a deeper understanding of their patterns and potential. The Feldenkrais Method, whether used in clinical settings, educational environments, or personal development situations, encourages people to explore the depths of their movement capabilities and discover new paths for growth and well-being.